Aberdeenshire

COUNCIL

Aberdeenshire Libraries
www.aberdeenshire.gov.uk/libraries
Renewals Hotline 01224 661511

Disclaimer: The information in this guide is not intended as a substitute for individual medical advice or treatment from your own doctor. If you are suffering from any health problems, it is important to consult a medical professional before following any of the advice or practices mentioned in this guide. While every attempt has been made to verify the information provided, neither the publisher nor the author can accept responsibility for any adverse effects or consequences resulting from the use of any of the preparations or procedures described. Research studies and institutions cited in this book should in no way be construed as an endorsement of anything in this guide.

Always consult your doctor before using any approaches or treatments mentioned in this publication if you are pregnant.

Medilance (Guernsey) Ltd
www.medilance.com

Contents

Chapter 2 Nutritional Approaches

Chapter 3 Nutritional Supplements

CHAPTER 1

Gallstone Essentials

Gallstones are one of the most common medical and surgical conditions, with as many as one in six people carrying them around in their gallbladder. Of those with gallstones, one in five will eventually experience colicky, upper abdominal pain as a result. The remaining four out of five 'carriers' may never know they harbour these potential pain-bombs, or may discover they own one or more as an incidental finding during routine health screening or investigations for another condition. Of those with 'silent' gallstones, the annual risk of going on to develop symptoms is estimated at around one in twenty-five.

Gallstones form when substances that are normally dissolved in your bile precipitate out to form solids, and can be thought of as bile solids.

Did you know? Thirty gallstones were found in the mummy of an Ancient Egyptian Priestess, dating from around 1500 BC.

1

What is bile?

Bile is a bitter, yellow-green fluid that is made in your liver and trickles down into your gallbladder for storage until needed. When your gallbladder contracts, bile flows down into the first part of your small intestines (duodenum). Here, it acts as a detergent, breaking down dietary fat globules into an emulsion of tiny droplets that are easier to absorb.

Every day, your liver produces between 750ml and 1500ml of bile. This yellow-green fluid consists of water, bile pigments (bilirubin and biliverdin), bile acid salts (sodium glycolate and sodium taurocholate), cholesterol and phospholipids such as lecithin (also known as phosphatidylcholine).

> *Did you know?* *Bile pigments are yellow (bilirubin) or green (biliverdin). Bacteria in your large bowel convert these to the more familiar brown colour found in faeces. If bile outflow from the liver is blocked, bilirubin will build up in your blood to cause jaundice and your faeces will develop a pale, putty colour.*

Your liver produces cholesterol from the saturated fats in your diet and secretes between 800mg and 1000mg into your bile on a daily basis. Normally, cholesterol is totally insoluble in water, but the lecithin and bile salts present in bile help to keep it dissolved.

How your gallbladder works

Your gallbladder is essentially a pear-shaped, storage pouch. A short cystic duct, two to four centimetres long, connects the gallbladder to your common bile duct. The lining of the cystic duct forms a series of undulating spiral folds that act like low-resistance valves to regulate bile flow in and out of your gallbladder. Muscle fibres within these folds relax or contract in response to various hormones, nerve impulses and certain drugs.

The flow of bile through the cystic duct is complex, and several studies show that bile can even flow in and out of the gallbladder at the same time. Between meals, your common bile duct mostly stays constricted while both your cystic duct and gallbladder relax. This causes a pressure gradient so that around seventy-five per cent of newly produced bile coming down from your liver is diverted into your gallbladder for storage. Some bile still trickles down into your duodenum, however.

Your gallbladder intermittently contracts and relaxes, rather like a bellows, even between meals. This stirs up the stored bile, just like laundry is occasionally churned during the rest-cycle of a washing machine. These contractions also sloosh bile to-and-fro within the cystic duct to prevent stagnation. Researchers believe these natural mechanisms help to prevent bile sludging to discourage gallstone formation.

3

During the night, and during other periods of fasting, your gallbladder only contracts strongly every few hours in response to nerve signals and an intestinal hormone called motilin (which causes intestinal contractions to move bowel contents onwards). As a result, your gallbladder regularly empties out 20% to 30% of its stored bile even when you are not eating.

The propulsive contractions of your gallbladder become progressively stronger during a meal. This is triggered in response to nerve impulses and other hormones secreted as food is churned within your stomach.

When semi-digested food passes from your stomach into the first part of your small intestines (duodenum) it triggers secretion of an intestinal hormone called cholecystokinin (CCK). This causes your gallbladder to contract fully, squirting 70% to 80% of its stored bile into the common bile duct and down into the duodenum. At the same time, CCK causes your pancreas to release powerful digestive enzymes into the duodenum to meet the newly arrived dietary fats, proteins and starches.

> *Did you know? The presence of gallstones affects how well your gallbladder contracts. Those classed as 'bad contractors' have severely impaired or even absent gallbladder emptying. Even 'good contractors' with gallstones may retain more bile after a meal, or when fasting, compared with normal, however. This retention of bile further adds to the growth of existing stones and the formation of new ones.*

As well as storing bile, your gallbladder reabsorbs some of the water present. While this makes bile more potent for breaking down dietary fats, it also increases the concentration of cholesterol and bile pigments present by three to five-fold. If the saturation balance tips the wrong way, dissolved substances can crystallise out of solution to form solid stones. This becomes increasingly likely if you make more cholesterol than usual or if more water is reabsorbed – for example if your gallbladder is not able to contract and empty itself properly so bile spends more time in storage.

NB If you don't have a gallbladder, bile trickles down into the duodenum continuously which sometimes causes problems such as bloating or loose bowels from poor digestion of dietary fats.

How do gallstones form?

The relative concentrations of water, bile salts, lecithin and cholesterol present in bile determine whether or not it becomes supersaturated, so that some of the dissolved substances fall out of solution. Imbalances leading to supersaturation may result from:

- Excessive secretion of cholesterol or bilirubin by the liver.
- Deficient secretion of bile salts or lecithin which are needed to make cholesterol soluble.
- Excessive production of gel-like mucus within the gallbladder.

- Bile staying in your gallbladder for long periods of time so more water is absorbed eg because of eating too little fat or not eating for extended periods of time so your gallbladder empties less frequently.
- Reduced ability of the gallbladder to contract between meals so that stored bile settles out or becomes 'stagnant'.
- Reduced or absent ability of the gallbladder to contract and empty at night, when biliary cholesterol saturation is highest because of lower bile salt secretion from the liver.

Bile crystallisation produces a gel-like suspension of cholesterol crystals or bilirubinate salts within your gallbladder, which is known as biliary sludge. These small crystals act as the seed around which gallstones can form. If your gallbladder empties normally, these tiny crystals may be ejected along with bile and flushed away. If your gallbladder emptying is impaired, however, these tiny grains may clump together, or slowly enlarge to form significant gallstones.

As the make-up of your bile changes on a daily basis, the growth of a gallstone is a stop-and-start process in which layers slowly build up – rather like a pearl grows around a grain of sand inside an oyster.

Seventy per cent of gallstones consist mainly of cholesterol in the form of cholesterol monohydrate crystals.

Up to thirty per cent of gallstones are mainly composed of bile pigments (in the form of calcium rubinate plus calcium carbonate and calcium phosphate).

What do gallstones look like?

Gallstones vary in size from one to 25 millimetres across. Some people develop one large stone, which may be as large as a golf ball, while others harbour up to 200 or more grit-like stones that resemble sandy gravel.

Cholesterol stones consist of at least 80% cholesterol by weight. Typically round or oval in shape, they are often large (two to three centimetres in length) and solitary. They also tend to be pale with a translucent appearance. Sometimes a ring of bile pigments or calcium salts may be deposited on their surface so they become pale yellow to dark green, or speckled like a quail's egg. Cholesterol stones are not easy to see on abdominal X-rays and are therefore described as 'radiolucent'.

Bile pigment stone are small, dark, crumbly, irregular in shape and contain less than 20% cholesterol. They are usually multiple and either black or brown in colour.

- Black pigment stones are rare in people under the age of 50, and may be associated with medical conditions that increase the rate at which haemoglobin (the red blood pigment) is broken down into bilirubin, or where reabsorption of the bilirubin in bile increases.

- Brown pigment stones are less common, and are associated with chronic infection of the bile ducts (cholangitis) with bacteria (eg Escherichia coli, Klebsiella) or in some countries with liver flukes or intestinal worms. These infections interact with bile lecithin to produce calcium fatty acid soaps that precipitate out within the bile ducts to form brown pigment stones.

Mixed stones contain between 20% and 80% cholesterol plus calcium salts, fatty acid salts and bile pigments. They are often multiple, faceted or squarish in shape and mottled in colour. Because of their calcium content, mixed stones show up on X-ray.

What causes gallstones?

A number of risk factors are associated with an increase chance of developing gallstones. Some risk factors may be improved significantly through diet and lifestyle changes. Others, such as increasing age, being female and having a strong family history are less easy to overcome.

Unmodifiable Risk Factors

- Age
- Female gender
- Heredity

Modifiable Risk Factors

- Obesity
- Rapid weight loss
- Poor diet
- Alcohol abstinence
- Smoking
- Lack of exercise
- Medical conditions
- Medications

Age

Gallstones become more likely as you get older. Although they are considered rare before the age of 20, the youngest girl to need her gallbladder and gallstones removed was only five years old.

Gallstones occurring in children are usually composed of bile pigments rather than cholesterol, and may relate to other medical conditions such as having thalassaemia or cystic fibrosis (see below).

> *Did you know? Ultrasound studies during pregnancy show that some foetuses develop gallstones, too, although little is known about how or why this happens. Treatment with bile acids usually helps them dissolve within 16 weeks of birth.*

9

Increasing age tends to be associated with rising cholesterol levels, reduced production of bile acids and less efficient contraction of the gallbladder, all of which predispose towards gallstones.

Some cholesterol becomes absorbed into the gallbladder lining, causing it to thicken and impairing its ability to relax and contract. Long-term exposure to bile acid salts, and possibly intestinal bacteria, may also set up a low-grade inflammatory or immune response which contributes to loss of gallbladder function and the development of gallstones.

However, it's now generally accepted that the main reason why increasing age is associated with an increased risk of gallstones is simply because it increases your exposure to all the other risk factors listed below.

Gender

Females are four times more likely to develop gallstones than men up until the age of 30 years, three times more likely between the ages of 30 and 40, twice as likely between the ages of 40 to 50, and around twenty percent more likely between the ages of 50 and 60. After this age, the incidence between males and females becomes similar.

Women are more prone to gallstones because of the effects of the female hormones, oestrogen and progesterone.

- Oestrogen stimulates a liver enzyme (HMG-CoA reductase – the same enzyme blocked by statin drugs) to increase cholesterol production.
- Progesterone has a relaxing effect on smooth muscle fibres which inhibits gallbladder contraction. This increases the chance of stored bile settling out to form a 'sludge' so that cholesterol or other ingredients are likely to precipitate out as stones.

Oestrogen and progesterone levels are especially high during pregnancy, and the occurrence of bile sludge tends to increase steadily as pregnancy progresses. This may explain why a woman's risk of developing gallstones increases with the more pregnancies she has. Studies have found, for example, that women who've had at least two pregnancies are four to twelve times more likely to develop gallstones than women of the same age and weight who've never had children.

The effects of progesterone wear off within a few weeks once a pregnancy ends, however, and biliary sludge usually disappears - as do some pregnancy-associated gallstones. However, gallstone crystals that have already started to seed may remain to grow bigger – especially during a subsequent pregnancy.

Heredity

Gallstones seem to 'run' in some families. The genes you inherit will affect the size and shape of your gallbladder, and the amount of cholesterol and bile acids your liver produces. Studies involving identical and non-identical twins (to compare nature versus nurture) suggest that around one third of your gallstone risk is inherited, which suggests that seventy per cent is down to other factors – especially your diet and lifestyle.

Obesity

If you carry excess weight, your risk of gallstones increases. A woman who is classed as obese (body mass index greater than 30 Kg/M^2) is twice as likely to develop gallstones as a similar woman in the healthy weight range for her height. Those who are morbidly obese (BMI greater than 40 Kg/M2) have a seven-fold increased risk. The risks are even higher for people who store excess fat around their waists rather than around their hips (central obesity). The reason for these links is partly due to unhealthy diet, and partly because obesity causes a low grade inflammation that increases cholesterol production in the liver. As a result, the longer you have been overweight, the higher your risk.

Children who are significantly overweight are also more likely to develop gallstones if they carry their weight problems into adult life.

Rapid weight loss

Perhaps surprisingly, rapid weight loss also increases your risk of gallstones. When you reduce the amount of food you eat, or follow a low-fat diet, less bile is squirted into your duodenum and more stays pooled in your gallbladder from which gallstones can precipitate.

A study involving almost 90,000 nurses found that losing between 4 kg and 10 kg weight over a two year period increased the risk of gallstone disease by 44% compared with women whose weight changed by less than 4 kg over the same period. Those who lost more than 10 kg were almost twice as likely to develop gallstone disease, with a 94% increased risk. Other studies show that losing more than 1.5 kg/week seems to dramatically increase the risks. And among patients who lose weight rapidly after bariatric surgery (eg fitting a 'lap band' to reduce stomach volume) more than one in four develop bile 'sludge' in the gallbladder during the first six weeks after their operation, and it's from this sludge that gallstones are likely to crystallise out.

Poor diet

A diet that is high in saturated fat and pre-formed cholesterol increases the amount of cholesterol that your liver pumps into your bile. If your diet is also low in fibre (which acts like a sponge to mop up fats) more cholesterol is absorbed back into your circulation from your intestines.

The opposite is also true - a diet that is unusually low in fat can promote gallstones as the gallbladder empties less frequently as it mainly contracts in response to dietary fats. Lack of vitamin C can also play a role, as vitamin C is needed to make the bile acids that keep cholesterol dissolved in your bile. Nutrition is covered more fully later in this guide.

Alcohol abstinence

A moderate intake of alcohol protects against gallstones through effects on liver cell metabolism and cholesterol balance. In particular, it increases production of 'good' HDL-cholesterol (which helps to protect against heart disease although there is no clear proof that it reduces the occurrence of cholesterol gallstones). Alcohol also acts as a solvent, helping to stop the components of gallstones precipitating out of solution in stored bile. This is probably the main way in which a moderate intake of alcohol reduces gallstone formation (but please don't use this as an excuse to increase your intake!)

Lack of exercise

Research shows that a low level of physical activity increases your risk of gallstones, while regular vigorous exercise, such as brisk walking, is protective. The more time you spend sitting every day, the higher your risk of gallstones.

Smoking

Some studies show a direct link between the number of cigarettes smoked and the risk of gallstone disease. Other studies have found no relationship. If there is a link, it is thought to relate to a combination of reduced liver production of 'good' HDL-cholesterol in smokers, and alterations in the production of gallbladder mucus as well as impaired gallbladder contraction.

Medical conditions

Some pre-existing medical conditions are associated with an increased risk of developing gallstones. These include:

* Hereditary hyperlipidaemia (in which blood triglyceride levels are significantly higher than normal).
* Cystic fibrosis (in which secretions such as bile are more sticky than normal).
* Any illness that increases the rate at which haemoglobin (the red blood pigment) is broken down into bilirubin (eg haemolytic anaemia, thalassaemia, sickle cell disease, malaria).
* Any illness that increases the reabsorption of bilirubin from your small bowel (eg ileal disease, bowel bypass or resection).

Interestingly, there is only a weak link between raised blood cholesterol levels and gallstones, perhaps because high circulating cholesterol levels reflect a reduced ability to secrete cholesterol into the bile.

Having type 2 diabetes appears to increase the risk of gallstones and a study from England found that gallstones were twice as common in people with diabetes. The link is thought to result from the associated metabolic changes that tend to raise your blood levels of triglyceride fat, cause fats to accumulate in your liver, promote obesity and reduce gallbladder contraction.

Type 2 diabetes is often preceded by a condition known as metabolic syndrome, or prediabetes, in which blood pressure and triglycerides are raised, the waistline is expanded by fat deposited around the internal organs, and glucose control is impaired. A study in China involving 7570 people found that men with metabolic syndrome were three times more likely to have gallstones than normal, while for women the risk was increased fivefold.

Infection of the bile ducts increases the risk of brown pigment stones. These are especially common in East Asia (eg Thailand, Vietnam, Cambodia) where parasitic liver flukes that target the gallbladder and bile ducts are ingested in raw or undercooked fish. The larvae of giant intestinal round worms (*Ascaris lumbricoides*) can also infect the bile ducts, or the calcified coat of their eggs may stimulate stone formation. Intestinal worm infections are ingested from food grown in soil fertilised with untreated sewage. An estimated one billion people are infected with these round worms worldwide, with the highest rates in China, Southeast Asia and Africa.

Medications

Some drug treatments increase the risk of gallstones by increasing cholesterol secretion into bile (eg clofibrate, oestrogen), by binding to bile acids (eg cholestyramine), by blocking gallbladder contraction (eg octreotide), by reducing gallbladder contraction (eg progesterones) or by triggering the formation of bile sludge (eg ceftriaxone).

Women on hormone replacement therapy (HRT) or hormonal methods of contraception also have a higher risk of gallstones as a result of their medication. Some studies suggest that using the oral contraceptive pill, or using HRT for two or more years, means you are at least three times more likely to develop gallstones than if you hadn't used them. This risk may be associated with inheriting certain genes, however, and may not apply to all women. However, the risk associated with modern low-dose contraceptive pills containing less than 50 micrograms of oestrogen plus one of the newer progestogens (such as desogestrel, drospirenone, norethindrone or levonorgestrel) may be small so that overall, they do not raise your chance of developing gallstones significantly.

What symptoms do gallstones cause?

Around seventy per cent of people with gallstones do not have symptoms at the time of diagnosis – the stones are discovered during routine check-ups or investigations for other conditions.

Larger stones that are not causing symptoms are often left alone as these tend to remain 'silent'. However, small gallstones have the potential to pass into your sensitive bile duct to cause pain (biliary colic) and may increase your risk of developing inflammation of the gallbladder (cholecystitis), inflammation of the pancreas (pancreatitis) or obstructive jaundice at a later date. Some surgeons therefore recommend gallbladder removal to prevent this.

Belching

Bringing up wind (burping) is common in people with gallbladder disease, some of whom let rip with impressively long and loud belches which are beyond their control and are socially embarrassing. The cause appears to be three fold:

- Poor digestion of fats due to reduced bile production (poor contraction of the gallbladder).
- Air swallowing when eating.
- Lack of stomach acid (hypochlorhydria).

Reduced production of stomach acid is commonly associated with gallstones. Although this does not seem to cause the gallstones in the first place, it may develop as a result of impaired gastric function in general (perhaps related to abnormal nervous or intestinal hormone responses) and to chronic cholecystitis (see below).

Taking digestive enzyme supplements and/or betaine hydrochloride capsules with meals may help to relieve belching (see Supplements section).

Try not to be embarrassed by belching. Just smile and say 'Sorry, it's not me but my gallbladder!'

Biliary colic

When you eat, your gallbladder contracts to squirt bile into your duodenum. When gallstones are present, contraction may push a stone into the spiral cystic duct that connects your gallbladder to your common bile duct. This disrupts bile flow and the bile duct muscles will contract continually in an attempt to force bile through. This sustained contraction, plus the stone grating against the sensitive cystic duct lining, causes a sudden onset of spasmodic pain. This typically occurs a couple of hours after eating when food passes from the stomach into the duodenum to trigger gallbladder contraction.

Spasm of the gallbladder and associated bile ducts causes a severe pain known as biliary colic. The pain usually begins suddenly across the upper abdomen – often after a fatty meal - and may be difficult to locate exactly. It may settle in the upper right-hand side of your abdomen, and spread to your upper back, between your shoulder blades, or just under your right shoulder blade. The severe pain tends to come and go in waves (colicky) but does not always fluctuate. Some people feel sick or vomit, and belching is

19

common. The 'attack' typically lasts from 15 minutes to two hours but can persist up to 24 hours. Once the pain goes away (either subsiding spontaneously or with the help of analgesics and anti-spasmodic medication) a mild aching or soreness may last for around one day.

If the gallstone is too big to pass further into the bile duct, it may settle back into your gallbladder, but symptoms may recur when your gallbladder contracts after eating fatty foods. This is sometimes referred to as having 'grumbling' gallstones. If the stone is small enough to pass into the bile duct, it may eventually travel down into the duodenum after a period of excruciating pain.

Acute cholecystitis

A small gallstone can become stuck in the cystic duct between your gallbladder and bile duct. It then acts like a valve stopper, allowing bile to enter but not to leave. When this happens, your gallbladder becomes increasingly distended with trapped bile and the resulting build-up of pressure leads to discomfort and inflammation (acute cholecystitis).

The main symptom of acute cholecystitis is continuous pain in your upper abdomen, either in the middle or on the right-hand side, which spreads through to your back or below your right shoulder blade. The pain may be sharp, cramping or dull and is usually steady, rather than the wave-like colicky pain associated with biliary colic. Usual treatment involves hospital bed rest, painkillers, remaining 'nil-by-mouth' and receiving fluids via an intravenous drip. This often allows the gallstone to drop back into the gallbladder so the inflammation and symptoms settle.

If the bile trapped behind the gallstone becomes infected, however, the pain is longer-lasting, more severe and associated with a fever, nausea and vomiting. The upper right-hand side of the abdomen will be tender when a doctor presses over the swollen, infected gallbladder. If not treated promptly, this can progress to sepsis - often referred to as septicaemia or blood poisoning - in which bacteria grow and multiply within the blood stream. Patients will feel very ill with fever, chills, rigors (shakes), a rapid pulse, rapid breathing, vomiting and they may even collapse with dangerously low blood pressure (septic shock).

Another complication of acute cholecystitis is perforation of the infected gallbladder so that bile, pus and even gallstones leak into the abdominal cavity. This will cause severe abdominal pain (peritonitis) and must be treated as a surgical emergency.

Although antibiotics will resolve an uncomplicated episode of acute cholecystitis infection, removal of the gallbladder (cholecystectomy) is normally also advised as the infection will almost inevitably recur. In patients who are very ill, a tube may be passed through the skin into the gallbladder to drain away pus and infected bile until they are well enough for surgery.

Chronic cholecystitis

Repeated attacks of acute (sudden) cholecystitis can lead to long-term (chronic) inflammation. The walls of the gallbladder thicken and the organ shrinks so that it becomes less and less able to concentrate, store or release bile. As further attacks of acute cholecystitis are almost inevitable, the gallbladder and the stones it contains are best removed.

Pancreatitis

Your pancreas lies beneath your stomach, nestled in the curve of the duodenum. It function as both an endocrine gland (secreting hormones such as insulin directly into the blood stream) and as an exocrine gland (secreting powerful digestive enzymes into the pancreatic duct).

Pancreatic digestive juices pass via the pancreatic duct to join the flow of bile at the base of the common bile duct. If a gallstone or biliary sludge blocks the outlet of your pancreatic duct, the powerful enzymes trickling down from your pancreas become trapped. This causes the pancreas to become inflamed, either suddenly (acute pancreatitis) or in a persistent, grumbling manner (chronic pancreatitis).

Pancreatitis is one of the most common diseases seen by gastroenterologists, accounting for one in fifty hospital admissions in Western countries. It is associated with gallstones, a high alcohol intake and having a raised triglyceride level (either from the genes you inherit or from excessive intakes of alcohol, fats or carbohydrates).

Overall, males are seven times more likely to develop pancreatitis than females. Many cases have no obvious cause, and as more of these cases occur in Spring than at any other time of the year, a viral infection may be involved (although if you have gallstones these are the primary suspects).

Pancreatitis is a serious condition requiring intensive care in hospital to maintain fluid and salt balance, and to keep blood pressure and glucose levels normal until the pancreas recovers.

Jaundice

If a gallstone blocks the flow of bile into the duodenum, your bowel motions will become pale and clay-like. Bilirubin will build up in your circulation to cause jaundice and the whites of your eyes will turn yellow while your urine becomes unusually dark. Your skin will develop an orange-yellow colour if the jaundice is severe.

What medical tests can help?

Gallstones are often found by chance when another condition is investigated. If you present with abdominal pain suggestive of gallstones, some routine screening blood tests are usually requested. You may also have a urine test (to rule out diabetes and to look for blood which may suggest you have kidney stones or an infection). A chest X-ray and heart tracing (ECG) may be requested to rule out other causes of upper abdominal/back pain such as pneumonia or a heart attack. Occasionally, gallstones can be seen on chest X-ray. The best and least invasive way to diagnose gallstones, however, is via an ultrasound.

Blood tests

A full blood count (FBC) will check for anaemia (associated with some pigment stones) and measure your level of white blood cells to show whether or not infection (eg cholecystitis) is present.

Liver function tests will show how well your liver is working, whether or not jaundice is present and, if so, whether this is due to blockage of bile outflow or to liver disease.

Liver function tests (LFTs) include measurements of:
Albumin - the main protein made by the liver; low levels suggest the liver is not functioning properly.
Alkaline phosphatase - an enzyme which mainly comes from the liver bile ducts (and bone). A raised level may indicate blocked bile ducts (or bone disease).
Alanine aminotransferase (ALT) - an enzyme which helps to process proteins in the liver; it is raised when the liver is inflamed (hepatitis).

<u>Aspartate transaminase</u> (AST) - another enzyme involved in processing proteins in the liver and in muscles. Raised levels may suggest problems with liver or muscle cells.

<u>Bilirubin</u> - a pigment produced by recycling haemoglobin from worn-out red blood cells. Liver cells process bilirubin by attaching it to a sugar to form conjugated bilirubin which is excreted into the bile ducts. A raised level of conjugated bilirubin can indicate that bile outflow is blocked by a gallstone. It can also be raised with hepatitis or long-term alcohol abuse. A raised level of unconjugated bilirubin occurs when there is an excessive breakdown of red blood cells - for example in haemolytic anaemia, which is associated with pigment gallstones.

<u>Gamma glutamyl transferase</u> (gammaGT) - a liver enzyme involved in breaking down alcohol and some drugs. A raised level can suggest a high alcohol intake, the side effects of medication, or liver damage, but the genes you inherit also affect how much gammaGT you make. If your gammaGT is raised but all other liver tests are normal, the result is usually of no consequence.

<u>Globulin</u> - a type of circulating blood protein made in the liver which is increased if inflammation or infection is present.

Ultrasound

A traditional, plain abdominal X-ray only picks up 10% of gallstones – those with a high calcium content. In contrast, an ultrasound scan can accurately detect 90% to 95% of gallstones.

Ultrasound scanning is a painless technique in which a probe is run up and down your abdomen. This passes inaudible, high frequency sound waves through your abdominal wall which bounce back from tissues of different density. Returning signals are analysed by computer and translated into a visual image. As well as identifying gallstones, ultrasound scanning can measure the diameter of your common bile duct and check that your liver and hepatic bile ducts look healthy. If your gallbladder wall shows thickening (greater than 3 mm) then cholecystitis is likely.

Ultrasound scanning may miss very tiny stones and those lodged in the bile duct system, of which only around half are identified with certainty. If a doctor suspects a gallstone is lodged in your bile duct (due to jaundice or abnormal liver function tests), ultrasound may be repeated after an interval to help identify a stone that was previously missed.

Computerised tomography (CT) can also be used to detect common bile duct stones.

Cholangiography

In the past, when a stone was thought to be lodged in the common bile duct, a special dye test called cholangiography was carried out. This involves injecting a special 'dye' into a vein which becomes concentrated in the bile and gallbladder system as it is excreted from the body. This 'dye' shows up on X-rays, outlining the gallbladder and bile ducts, and revealing any stones as black 'holes' or filling defects where the dye is absent.

Laparoscopic ultrasonography (in which telescopic instruments are inserted through the abdominal wall under general anaesthetic) has now replaced cholangiography as the method of choice for detecting common bile duct stones as it is more accurate and safer.

ERCP

Endoscopic retrograde cholangiopancreatography (a mouthful usually shortened to ERCP) involves injecting a 'dye' into the lower end of the common bile duct via a fine catheter that is passed down through your mouth and stomach into the duodenum. The 'dye' enters the bile duct to reveal stones as non-filling shadows when X-rayed.

ERCP has the advantage of allowing instrumental removal of a trapped bile duct stone as part of the procedure. It does increase the risk of introducing infection into the bile ducts to cause cholangitis, however.

Cholescintigraphy

A scan of the liver and bile ducts, known as cholescintigraphy, may be performed to reveal a blocked cystic duct. A radioactive chemical or tracer 'dye' is injected into a vein in your arm and becomes concentrated within the bile as it is excreted from your body. A nuclear medicine scanner (gamma camera) can then track the flow of tracer from your liver into your gallbladder and duodenum. Normally, the trace arrives within the gallbladder within an hour of injection. If the gallbladder is not visualised within four hours, this suggests that bile cannot pass in and out of your cystic duct (due to a gallstone blockage) or that your gallbladder is not functioning (cholecystitis).

Deciding how to treat your gallstones

Your main treatment options are:

- **Conservative care** in which you manage your symptoms through nutritional and lifestyle changes to help prevent gallstone pain.
- **Medical approaches** such as pain killers and antispasmodic medication when necessary. It is sometimes also possible to dissolve gallstones with medicines to reduce their size or even melt them away, although they often recur.
- **Surgery** to remove your gallbladder.

Which option you choose initially will depend on the severity and frequency of your symptoms and your overall general health. If your gallstones were diagnosed by chance, and have never caused symptoms, you may wish to avoid surgery. In this case, nutritional and lifestyle approaches help between 85% and 90% of people have no further problems, so they live quite happily with their well-behaved stones. Between 10% and 25% will eventually develop symptoms, however, and may then decide to investigate medical approaches or proceed to surgery.

CHAPTER 2

Nutritional Approaches

If you wish to avoid surgery, you may need to make significant changes to your diet and lifestyle, as your current eating habits and way of life have not stopped your gallstones from developing.

Lose any excess weight slowly

Being overweight or obese increases your risk of gallstones – it is estimated that 38% of symptomatic gallstones are directly associated with having a Body Mass Index of more than 25.

Body Mass Index is calculated by dividing your weight (in kilograms) by the square of your height (in metres):

BMI = your weight (Kg) divided by [your height (M) x your height (M)].

BMI calculators are widely available on-line to save you having to work this out for yourself.

Your BMI results will put you in one of four different weight bands, which are defined by the Word Health Organisation as follows:

BMI	WEIGHT BAND
Up to 18.5	Underweight
18.5 - 24.9	Healthy weight
25 - 29.9	Overweight
30 and over	Obese

Ideally, you want a BMI of between 18.5 and 24.9 kg/M^2 as this puts you in the healthy weight range for your height. You can find the ideal weight range for your height in the table below (calculations rounded up or down as appropriate).

Height		Healthy Weight Range	
Metres	Feet	Kg	Stones
1.47	4'10"	40.0 - 53.8	6st 4lb – 8st 6lb
1.50	4'11"	41.6 - 56.0	6st 8lb – 8st 11lb
1.52	5ft	42.7 - 57.5	6st 10 – 9st
1.55	5'1"	44.4 – 59.8	7st – 9st 5lb
1.57	5'2"	45.6 – 61.4	7st 2lb – 9st 9lb
1.60	5'3"	47.4 – 63.7	7st 6lb – 10st
1.63	5'4"	49.2 – 66.2	7st 10lb – 10st 5lb
1.65	5'5"	50.4 – 66.6	7st 13lb – 10st 7lb

1.68	5'6"	52.2 – 70.3	8st 3lb – 11st
1.70	5'7"	53.5 - 72.0	8st 6lb – 11st 4lb
1.73	5'8"	55.4 – 74.5	8st 10lb – 11st 10lb
1.75	5'9"	56.7 - 76.3	8st 13lb – 12st
1.78	5'10"	58.6 – 78.9	9st 3lb – 12st 5lb
1.80	5'11"	60.0 - 80.7	9st 6lb – 12st 9lb
1.83	6 ft	62.0 - 83.4	9st 10lb – 13st 1lb
1.85	6'1"	63.3 – 85.2	9st 13lb – 13st 5lb
1.88	6'2"	65.4 – 88.0	10st 4lb – 13st 11lb
1.90	6'3"	66.8 - 89.9	10st 7lb – 14st 1lb
1.93	6'4"	68.9 – 92.8	10st 12lb – 14st 8lb

If you need to lose weight, it is important to do so at a slow, steady rate and to avoid crash dieting.

Rapid weight loss of more than two or three pounds per week appears to promote the development of gallstones and increases the risk that silent gallstones start to cause symptoms. This is partly linked with changes in bile composition, so that the relative amount of cholesterol present increases compared with the amount of bile salts present – as a result, less cholesterol stays dissolved. At the same time, cutting back on eating reduces gallbladder contractions so stored bile becomes more static and prone to 'sludging'.

Which weight loss diet is best?

People with gallstones were traditionally advised to follow a low-fat, high fibre diet. Low fat was recommended to reduced gallbladder contractions so that small gallstones are less likely to get pushed into the mouth of the spiral duct. However, a diet that is too low in fat may have the opposite effect, as delayed gallbladder emptying leads to bile stasis so that stones are be more likely to form. Eating healthy fats is therefore beneficial and a Mediterranean-style weight loss diet that contains healthy fats (such as those found in olive oil, nuts and oily fish) along with plenty of fruit and vegetables (rich in vitamin C and other antioxidants plus fibre) is more beneficial.

> *Dietary factors that appear to increase your risk of developing cholesterol gallstones include consuming excess cholesterol-rich foods, saturated fat, trans fatty acids and carbohydrate, especially refined sugars.*

Eat more monounsaturated fats

Monounsaturated fats consist of chains of carbon atoms in which there is only one double (unsaturated) bond.

Monounsaturated fats are beneficial for general health as they are metabolised in a way that lowers your level of 'bad' LDL-cholesterol while having a neutral effect on your 'good' HDL-cholesterol. Olive, macadamia nut, and avocado oils are all rich sources of mono-unsaturated fats and their beneficial effect on blood cholesterol balance may help to reduce gallstone formation while promoting healthy contraction of your gallbladder.

As a bonus, a diet high in monounsaturates helps to reduce your risk of hardening and furring up of the arteries (atherosclerosis), high blood pressure, coronary heart disease and stroke. This is thought to explain some of the benefits of the Mediterranean diet.

Eat more omega-3 polyunsaturated fats

Polyunsaturated fats consist of chains of carbon atoms in which there are two or more double (unsaturated) bonds. The way your body handles these fats depends on where the double bonds are found.

- If the first double bond involves the third carbon atom, the molecule is classed as an omega-3 fatty acid.
- If the first double bond involves the sixth carbon atom, it is classed as an omega-6 fatty acid.

Omega-3 fatty acids (especially the long-chain DHA and EPA found in fish oils) are converted into substances that reduce inflammation. This helps to balance the action of omega-6 fatty acids (derived from vegetables oils such as corn, sunflower and safflower oils) which are known to promote inflammation.

To reduce gallbladder inflammation, whether from food sensitivity (see later) or gallstone inflammation, it's best to consume more omega-3 fats (eg found in flaxseed, walnut and fish oils). These may help to protect against gallstone formation. In one small study, seven people with cholesterol gallstones took high doses of omega-3 fish oils (11.3g fish oils supplying 3.75g omega-3s) per day. This lowered the cholesterol saturation of their bile by twenty-five per cent to reduce the risk of more cholesterol precipitating out.

Fish with the highest content of beneficial omega-3s include kippers, salmon, mackerel, pilchards, herring, fresh (but not tinned) tuna and sardines.

To reduce your intake of inflammatory omega-6s aim to consume fewer:

- Omega-6 rich vegetable oils such as safflower oil, grape-seed oil, sunflower oil, corn oil, cottonseed oil or soybean oil (replace with rapeseed, olive or walnut oils).
- Margarines based on omega-6 oils such as sunflower or safflower oil.
- Bought convenience foods.
- Fast-foods.
- Manufactured goods such as cakes, sweets and pastries.

Eat more fibre

Fibre offers important protection against a number of long-term health problems, including gallstones. Soluble fibre such as pectins (eg found in apples, carrots) and gums (found in oat bran and beans) bind to cholesterol and bile salts in the gut to reduce their re-absorption. Bran fibre also has an effect on intestinal bacteria in the large bowel, so that when they break down bile acids, they produce less deoxycholic acid – a secondary bile acid that is reabsorbed to make the bile more conducive to gallstone formation. Research shows that adding 10g to 50g fibre supplements to your diet every day can lower the cholesterol saturation of bile within four to six weeks.

Researchers from Harvard looked for any association between fibre intake and the risk of cholecystectomy in almost 70,000 women, aged from 35 to 61 years, who were followed for 16 years. After taking all other risks factors into account, they found that women with the highest fibre intake were 13% less likely to undergo surgical removal of their gallbladder than those with the lowest fibre intake. Every 5g increase in total fibre intake reduced the risk by around 6% on average, with insoluble fibre proving more protective than soluble fibre. For those who ate the most fruit and vegetables (a major source of insoluble fibre), the risk of needing a gallbladder removal was 21% lower than those eating the least. Green leafy vegetables, citrus and other vitamin C-rich fruits and vegetables were most protective, along with cruciferous vegetables (members of the cabbage family).

Aim to eat at least five servings of fruit, vegetables and salad stuff per day – and preferably eight to ten – as well as eating more fibre-rich grains such as oats. Try porridge or unsweetened oatmeal-based muesli for breakfast, mix rolled oats into yogurts and eat oatcakes as a snack (topped with delicious nut omega-3 rich nut butters).

Eat more vegetable protein

A plant-based diet provides high levels of fibre, antioxidants (especially vitamin C) and plant sterols (substances that block cholesterol absorption) which all help to protect against gallstones. As a result, only one in eight female vegetarians develop gallstones compared with one in four women who do not follow a plant-based diet.

If you like meat, the good news is that just increasing your intake of fruit and vegetables, without cutting back on meat, also has a protective effect as vegetable protein in itself appears to inhibit gallstone formation. In particular, soy protein has a beneficial effect on cholesterol synthesis in the liver, the concentration of cholesterol in the bile, and the rate at which cholesterol crystals precipitate out of bile.

A US study that followed over 80,700 female nurses for twenty years found that, after taking other risk factors into account, women with the highest vegetable protein intake were 21% less likely to need their gallbladder surgically removed than those with the lowest intake. The amount of animal protein and total protein they ate did not significantly affect these results, suggesting that any increased consumption of vegetable protein can reduce the risk of cholecystectomy in women.

Eat more nuts

Nuts provide healthy polyunsaturated fats, monounsaturated fats, fibre, vitamins, minerals, antioxidants and plant sterols. Eating more nuts is known to have beneficial effects on cholesterol balance, and may help to help protect against cholesterol gallstones.

A US study that followed over 80,700 female nurses for twenty years found that women who ate nuts five or more times per week (including peanuts, which are really a legume, and peanut butter) were 34% less likely to need their gallbladder surgically removed than those who rarely or never ate nuts. When other factors were taken into account, such as saturated fat intake, weight, smoking status, alcohol and caffeine consumption, eating nuts at least five times a week appeared to lower the chance of needing a cholecystectomy by 15%. As a healthy snack, nuts and nut butters are certainly ones to go for.

Cut back on cholesterol-rich foods

Cholesterol is a fatty substance made in animal livers. The amount of cholesterol you obtain from your diet depends on the amount of animal-based products you eat. Studies show that the more cholesterol you eat, the more cholesterol is secreted into your bile. If the amount present (cholesterol saturation) is greater than can be maintained in solution, some cholesterol will precipitate out. This may trigger the formation of new gallstones, or enlarge any that are already present.

Typical diets provide between 500mg to 1000mg cholesterol per day. Some of the richest food sources of cholesterol are shown in the following table:

Food	Cholesterol per 100g
Pig liver	700 mg
Lamb kidney	610 mg
Caviar	588 mg
Lamb liver	400 mg
Chicken egg (whole, raw)	391mg
Chicken liver	350 mg
Calf liver	330 mg

Prawns	280 mg
Pheasant meat	220 mg
Butter	213 mg
Squid	200 mg
Duck meat	110mg
Lobster meat	110 mg
Hard cheese	100 mg
Lean beef	58 mg
Chicken meat	105 mg (dark meat)
	70 mg (white meat)

If you are advised to follow a low-cholesterol diet, you may be told to limit your daily intake to no more than 300mg per day – about the amount found in the yolk of a single large hen's egg.

However, most of the cholesterol in your circulation is made in your own liver, which produces around 800mg cholesterol every day from certain saturated fats in your diet.

Ideally, saturated fats should supply no more than 7% to 10% of your energy intake, which, for most people, means cutting back. Replace them with more beneficial monounsaturated fatty acids (found in olive, rapeseed, macadamia and avocado oils) or omega-3 polyunsaturated fats (found in fish, flaxseed and walnuts oils).

Cut back on carbohydrates – especially sugar

People who eat the most refined sugar (eg sucrose, fructose) have a higher than normal risk of developing gallstones, even if they are not overweight as a result of their dietary habits.

Experimental models suggest that if dietary sugar is replaced with starch, then the weight of gallstones produced would be expected to halve in females. This was tested in 13 volunteers with cholesterol gallstones who followed either a refined carbohydrate diet (including sugar and white flour) or an unrefined diet (wholegrains) for six weeks then swapped to the opposite diet. The cholesterol saturation of their bile was significantly higher on the refined carbohydrate diet than with the unrefined carbohydrate diet (a 25% difference). This suggests that following a wholegrain, unrefined carbohydrate diet may help to reduce the risk of further gallstone formation.

However, it is important not to consume too much carbohydrate – even if it is in the form of healthy wholegrains. Excess dietary carbohydrates are themselves converted into saturated fat in your liver for storage and these saturated fats can, in turn, be converted on to cholesterol and contribute to the gallstone formation.

Researchers from Harvard followed almost 70,000 women aged from 35 to 61 years for 16 years and looked at their diet and their risk of a variety of health problems. After taking all other risks factors into account, they found that women with the highest carbohydrate intake were 35% more likely to undergo removal of their gallbladder than those with the lowest carbohydrate intake.

Overall, there is good supporting evidence that cutting back on carbohydrates in general, and following a low glycaemic diet in particular, helps to protect against gallstone disease.

What is a low glycaemic diet?

A food's glycaemic index shows how much it affects your blood glucose levels when compared with eating a known amount (50g) of glucose which is given an arbitrary GI value of 100. A food that raises blood glucose levels half as much as glucose therefore has a GI value of 50.

Foods with a high GI (70 or above) have a rapid effect on blood glucose levels.

Foods with a medium GI (56-69) produce a more sustained effect on blood glucose levels.

Foods with a low GI (less than 55) contain few carbohydrates, or carbohydrates that break down very slowly to produce only a minor effect on blood glucose levels.

Very low GI foods, with a value of less than 30, include butter, cheese, eggs, fish, grapefruit, green vegetables, meat, nuts, plums, seafood and pulses such as soy beans and kidney beans.

> **Did you know?** *Fructose sugar has a surprisingly low GI value of 23, as it must be converted into glucose in the liver before it can affect blood glucose levels.*

Glycaemic Index is not always helpful, however, as it is based on volunteers eating whatever quantity of food contains 50g of digestible carbohydrate. In the case of carrots, which contain only 7% carbohydrate, this involves eating several bunches, which is not a realistic amount!

Another system, the Glycaemic Load (GL) was therefore developed to take into account the amount of carbohydrate present in a typical portion. Glycaemic load is calculated by multiplying a food's glycaemic index by the amount of carbohydrate found in a serving, then dividing the result by 100. This provides more useful information as, for example, an average serving of white pasta contains more than 50g digestible carbohydrate and has a larger impact on blood glucose levels than you might expect from its GI value alone.

A GL value of 20 or more is classed as High, a GL of 11 to 19 is classed as Medium while values of 10 or less are classed as Low.

In general, you may eat foods with a low GL value freely, but should aim to moderate your intake of foods with a moderate GL value, and take care not to eat too many foods with a high GL.

LOW GL Eat reasonably freely in a varied diet

Sweetcorn, boiled	Mixed grain bread
Wholemeal bread	Apples
Muesli	Oranges
Wholemeal rye bread	Pears
Grapes	Peas
Chickpeas	Carrots
Mango	Whole Milk
Fresh pineapple	Cashew nuts
Kidney beans, cooked	Raw cherries
Kiwi fruit	Peanuts

MODERATE GL Go easy, select small portions

Brown rice, boiled	Banana
White spaghetti, boiled	Unsweetened orange juice
Wholemeal spaghetti, boiled	Parsnips
New potatoes, boiled	Sweet potato
Porridge	Unsweetened apple juice
Bulgur wheat	Honey

HIGH GL Keep your intake to a minimum

Raisins	White rice, boiled
Baked potato	Cornflakes

As most fruit and vegetables (excluding potatoes) are not major contributors to carbohydrate intake, they have a relatively low glycaemic index/load and do not normally need to be restricted. Take care with dried fruit, such as raisins, however, whose sugars are concentrated due to the evaporation of water.

Did you know? *Glycaemic index and load values for almost 2000 foods can be found at www.glycemicindex.com courtesy of the University of Sidney.*

You can have coffee – in moderation!

The caffeine in coffee stimulates liver function and increases bile flow to reduce your risk of gallstones. Men who drink two or more cups of coffee per day are 40 % to 45% less likely to develop gallstone symptoms than non-coffee drinkers. For women, the risk is reduced by 22% to 28%. The same benefits are not seen with decaffeinated coffee, suggesting that caffeine is the active ingredient.

A study of 2417 people who filled out a dietary questionnaire and underwent ultrasound screening for gallstones found that caffeine consumption was associated with a 23% lower risk of having gallstones. Surprisingly, this result was not deemed statistically significant, but it is suggestive of a protective effect and certainly doesn't increase the risk.

Don't overdo coffee intake, however. Excess caffeine can mimic the stress response to cause jitters, irritation and anxiety. Suddenly cutting back a high intake can also lead to withdrawal symptoms including headache. Cut back slowly and aim to have no more than two or three caffeinated drinks per day.

You can have alcohol - in moderation!

Alcohol is an excellent solvent and, in moderation, may help to protect against gallstones.

When healthy volunteers who rarely consumed alcohol started to drink 39 g alcohol (equivalent to 3-4 drinks daily) for six weeks, the cholesterol saturation of their bile reduced, which would be expected to protect against gallstone formation.

A study of over 25,000 men and women living in Norfolk found that every unit of alcohol consumed per week decreased the risk of gallstone symptoms by 3% in men, but had no effect in women. Other studies have also found an inverse association between alcohol intake and gallstones so that the more someone drank, the more their risk of gallstones reduced. However, this may be partly explained by the fact that people with gallstone symptoms often cut back on alcohol use or avoid it altogether. When this effect was taken into account, the presumed protective effect of alcohol against gallstones disappears.

In excess, alcohol damages your liver and increases the risk of pancreatitis – especially when gallstones are present – and may even increase the risk of developing gallstone symptoms.

A large study looking at over 100,000 people found that gallstones were diagnosed in 5.2% of those without liver disease, in 9.1% with alcoholic fatty liver and in 9.5% of people with alcoholic liver cirrhosis. This suggests that excess consumption of alcohol may almost double the risk of gallstone symptoms.

Best advice is to stick to within recommended alcohol intakes of no more than 2 to 3 units per day (14 units per week total) for women or 3 to 4 units per day (21 units per week total) for men.

> *Did you know? A unit of alcohol is equivalent to 10ml or 8 grams of pure alcohol. Half a pint (300ml) of beer, lager or cider that is 3.5% alcohol in strength contains one unit. But many lagers now contain 5% and some versions supply as much as 9% alcohol. One small (100ml) glass of wine that is 10% alcohol in strength contains one unit, but most wines are now much stronger (12% to 15% alcohol) and come in 250ml glasses. Depending on its % alcohol, a bottle of wine typically contains between 8 and 11 units of alcohol. A 25ml pub measure of 40% spirit contains one unit, but many outlets now serve 35ml measures as standard, and will often serve a double unless you specify a single. To calculate how much you are drinking, use the handy unit calculator at www.drinkaware.co.uk.*

The Role Of Food Allergies And Intolerances

Some researchers have suggested that the symptoms of gallstone disease may partly relate to unrecognised reactions to food.

A classic food allergy involves a type of antibody called IgE which causes the rapid onset of potentially serious symptoms including swelling of the face, difficulty breathing and even collapse (anaphylactic shock). Less serious reactions due to food intolerances tend to come on more slowly and may be delayed for hours or even days after eating the culprit substance. These reactions involve immune cells which, it is suggested, may infiltrate the gallbladder wall causing swelling, increased mucus secretion and reduced contraction as a result of an 'allergic' cholecystitis.

This theory is supported by a small trial involving six people with untreated coeliac disease (intolerance to gliadin, a protein found in gluten), six normal volunteers and six people whose coeliac disease was being successfully treated with a gluten-free diet. After an overnight fast, all drank a liquid fat meal and their gallbladder emptying was monitored to determine how long it took for half the bile in their gallbladder to be ejected as a result of natural gallbladder contraction. This took around twenty minutes in both the normal volunteers and in those with treated coeliac disease. For those with untreated coeliac disease, however, it took 154 minutes for the gallbladder to empty by half. The researchers concluded that untreated coeliac disease (gliadin intolerance) causes a reversible defect of gallbladder emptying, and that this is linked with delayed release of cholecystokinin (CCK, the intestinal hormone that triggers gallbladder contraction).

Little research has occurred in this area, however, with only one study from the 1940s putting 69 people with gallstones onto an elimination diet to look for food intolerances. They were initially allowed to eat beef, rye, soy, rice, cherries, peaches, apricots, beets and spinach with no restriction of fat intake. Within a week, all were symptom free. New foods were then reintroduced, one at a time, to see which retriggered their symptoms, if any. This study found that eggs triggered symptoms in 93% of patients. Other common culprits were pork (64%), onions (52%), chicken (35%), milk (25%), coffee (22%), oranges (19%), corn, beans and nuts (each 15%). Six percent of participants reacted to apples and/or tomatoes.

Everyone has a different profile of foods which may trigger their symptoms, however, and the only way to find out if this approach may help you is to follow an elimination diet. Although this approach may help to reduce gallstone symptoms, it will not dissolve any gallstones already present.

How to follow an elimination diet

The simplest type of elimination diet involves avoiding suspect foods until your symptoms have settled, then to sequentially re-introduce them, one at a time every three or four days, to identify any that bring on your gallstone symptoms. The foods to test are initially identified by keeping a food and symptom diary for at least one week.

A more advanced approach involves following a bland, hypoallergenic diet that initially allows you to eat only a few limited items, typically:

Grains: White rice, tapioca
Fruits: Pears, pear juice, cranberries
Vegetables: Squash, carrots, parsnips, lettuce, lentils, split peas
Meat: lamb, wild game, turkey

After symptoms have disappeared, you start to re-introduce eliminated foods one by one, usually at three day intervals, while keeping a careful food and symptom diary to help identify problem foods. If symptoms occur, you continue to avoid the test food and wait 48 hours after all symptoms have improved before testing another food.

A strict elimination and challenge diet is best carried out under the supervision of a nutritional therapist. This approach is time consuming and difficult to stick to, however.

IgG blood tests

These private tests look for raised blood levels of IgG antibodies against specific foods in an attempt to more easily identify those to which you are intolerant.

The measurement of food allergen-specific IgG antibodies requires a small, pin-prick sample of blood which you send off to a laboratory. Test kits to take the sample are available from many pharmacies and on-line. Your blood is subjected to sophisticated ELISA (Enzyme-Linked Immunosorbent Assay) testing that identifies the presence of raised levels of IgG antibody against over 100 individual food antigens.

Avoiding foods to which you have a raised IgG titre may improve gallstone symptoms in some people, but clinical trials have not yet been carried out to confirm this.

The Gallbladder Flush

The gallbladder or liver flush is a folk remedy said to promote the passage of gallstones. The 'flush' typically involves fasting for twelve hours and then drinking a large amount of olive oil and lemon juice. Usually, a laxative (eg Epsom salts) and/or an enema is also included. This regime produces diarrhoea, abdominal pain and the passage of multiple green, brown, yellow or black spheres which resemble gallstones.

However, analysis shows that these hardened blobs are not stones, but bile-stained 'soaps' produced by an interaction (saponification) between the ingested oil and other ingredients of the flush. They are often produced in quantities far greater than could be stored within a gallbladder, and can be told apart from real stones because the soap blobs:

- Are soft, waxy or gelatinous while real gallstones are either hard or dry and crumbly (friable) in texture.
- Float on toilet water as they are largely composed of oil, whereas genuine gallstones would sink.
- Do not have the sharp facets produced when real gallstones rub against each other in the gallbladder.
- Can be cut cleanly with a knife (unlike real gallstones) and often have a bright green translucency that is never seen with real stones.
- Disintegrate over time unless frozen, whereas gallstones are stable.

There is no scientific evidence that the gallbladder flush works, and it may in fact be harmful. Even if the large amount of oil did promote ejection of a small gallstone into the cystic duct and out into the bile duct, this would be immensely painful, debilitating and would probably involve admission to hospital for investigations and pain relief.

CHAPTER 3

Nutritional Supplements

A number of nutritional and herbal supplements may help to reduce the formation or enlargement of gallstones, though few if any are likely to dissolve them away.

Vitamin C

Vitamin C (ascorbic acid) is a water-soluble vitamin which cannot be stored in the body. A regular intake is therefore essential from your diet. Food sources include most fruit and vegetables, especially lemon, limes, oranges and other citrus fruit, berries, blackcurrants, capsicum peppers, kiwi fruit and green leafy vegetables.

Vitamin C is an important antioxidant in all body tissues, and protects cholesterol in the circulation from oxidation. It is essential for collagen production for healthy tissues, and contributes to immunity, energy production, nerve function and mood.

Importantly for those with cholesterol gallstones, it boosts production of bile acids and helps keep cholesterol dissolved in the bile.

In a 12 month trial, taking 500 mg vitamin C per day significantly lowered both cholesterol and triglyceride levels compared with inactive placebo. The researchers suggested that vitamin C helped to boost the liver's ability to convert cholesterol into bile acids which were then flushed from the body in the bile. Vitamin C does this by acting as a vital cofactor for an enzyme (7 alpha-hydroxylase) that determines the rate at which cholesterol is converted to bile acids – when vitamin C is lacking, the conversion slows. Bile acids are important for keeping unconverted cholesterol dissolved in bile and this is another of the many ways in which a vegetarian diet - typically high in vitamin C - helps to protect against gallstones.

Another interesting study investigated the effects of vitamin C on gallstones and bile composition in 16 people booked to undergo laparoscopic cholecystectomy. For two weeks before surgery, they took vitamin C at a dose of 500 mg, four times a day (ie 2g daily in total). The relative concentrations of cholesterol, bile acids and cholesterol concentration in their bile did not differ but bile acid composition significantly changed to contain a lower percentage of cholic acid and higher percentages of deoxycholic, ursodeoxycholic and lithocholic acids. The time for cholesterol to precipitate out of bile samples (nucleation time) became significantly longer than in similar patients who did not take vitamin C (7 days versus 2 days). This study strongly suggests that regular use of vitamin C supplements can help to reduce cholesterol gallstone formation.

Researchers then looked at the dietary habits of 7042 women and 6088 men in the US who completed national nutritional and health surveys between 1988 and 1994. Overall, 11% of the women and 4% of the men went on to report symptoms of gallstones or underwent cholecystectomy. When vitamin C intakes and blood levels were assessed, women with the highest vitamin C blood levels were the least likely to develop gallbladder disease. A similar relationship was not seen among men – possibly because of the lower numbers affected.

A similar study in Germany, involving both men and women, found that taking vitamin C supplements reduced the risk of gallstone disease by 66%. Out of 232 people who regularly took vitamin C supplements, only 11 (4.7%) developed gallstones compared with 156 of 1897 who did not take vitamin C supplements (8.2%).

Dose:

The EU RDA for vitamin C is 80 mg. An expert scientific panel in the US suggested that the intake needed to meet the requirement of half the healthy individuals in a population is 100 mg/day, and with a safety margin proposed a daily amount of 120 mg/day. The recommendation is 100mg per day in Austria, Germany and Switzerland.

Average dietary intakes from fruit and vegetables are around 64mg per day, with vegetarians often obtaining 200mg per day or more. Supplement doses above 3000mg per day (3g) can cause indigestion and diarrhoea. Diarrhoea has been reported in a few individuals at lower doses of 1000mg (1g), although this can be avoided by using the 'body ready' form known as ester C, which is more readily absorbed and used. Because of this, the upper safe level for long-term use from supplements is suggested as 1000mg (1 gram). It is a safe supplement, however, with a low incidence of adverse effects at doses of up to 3g daily.

Absorption and metabolism of vitamin C varies depending on the amount consumed. At intakes of up to 200 mg/day as a single dose, absorption of vitamin C is almost complete through an active transport process. At single doses of over 500 mg, it is also absorbed through a process of diffusion, but efficiency of absorption declines so that only half of a 1.5g dose is absorbed (ie 750mg), and only 16% of a 12g dose (ie just under 2 g is absorbed). So, if taking higher doses, break it down into lower doses spread throughout the day.

The dose used in the trial mentioned above, of 500mg four times a day, could be used to help prevent further gallstone formation.

Note: When taking vitamin C supplements, it is important to know that:

- High doses of vitamin C can affect the results of some urine tests, so inform your doctor that you are taking supplements whenever a urine sample is requested.
- Some urine test kits used to monitor diabetes are affected by high dose vitamin C – use a kit that is not affected.
- High-dose vitamin C may mask the presence of blood in stool tests – inform your doctor if you are advised to have one of these.
- People with iron-storage disease (haemochromatosis) should only take vitamin C supplements under medical advice.
- People with recurrent kidney stones may have a defect in ascorbic acid or oxalate metabolism, and should restrict daily vitamin C intakes to no more than 100 mg under medical advice.

If taking high-doses (above 2g per day), and you decide to cut back, do so slowly over a few weeks rather than stopping suddenly, in order to avoid a so-called 'rebound scurvy' effect. A sudden reduction in blood vitamin C concentration means that enzymes activated by high levels of vitamin C are suddenly deprived of the extra vitamin C they need to work properly, and this can produce temporary symptoms of vitamin C deficiency.

Magnesium

Magnesium is the fourth most common metal found in the body, with most (70%) stored in the bones and teeth. It is needed for over 300 enzymes to work properly in the body, and is involved in every major metabolic reaction from the synthesis of protein and genetic material to the processing of cholesterol, triglycerides, essential fatty acids, insulin and glucose.

One of the most important functions of magnesium is to maintain the integrity of the ion pumps that control flow of sodium, potassium, calcium, chloride and other salt components across cell membranes. By moving ions against gradients, these pumps allow cells to hold an electrical charge, nerve cells to pass electrical messages from one neurone to another, and muscle cells to contract. Magnesium is therefore essential for good gallbladder function.

Magnesium is obtained from eating beans (especially soy), nuts, whole grains (though once processed they lose most of their magnesium content), seafood and dark green, leafy vegetables. Chocolate, drinking water in hard-water areas, mineral seasoning salts and Brewer's yeast are also important sources.

Lack of magnesium affects an estimated one in ten people. A magnesium-deficient diet has been found to raise blood triglyceride levels and to lower 'good' HDL-cholesterol which might be expected to increase the risk of gallstones or gallstone symptoms.

This was confirmed in a study that followed over 42,700 male health professionals for fifteen years in the US. Men with the highest magnesium intake from food (greater than 409mg per day) were 33% less likely to develop gallstone disease than those with the lowest intake (less than 288mg per day). When other factors were taken into account (such as age, weight, smoking, exercise, medication, alcohol, fibre) the protective effect was only slightly reduced to a 28% lower relative risk. Another study from Spain also found that people with gallstones had a lower magnesium intake than those without gallstones.

Dose:

The EU RDA for magnesium is 375mg daily. Average UK intakes are 280mg from food, plus 100mg per day from drinking water in some areas. The upper safe limit for long-term use from supplements is suggested as 400mg per day.

Note:
- Excess magnesium can produce a laxative action (a sometimes desirable effect for which Epsom salts are commonly used).

Lecithin

Lecithin, also known as phosphatidylcholine, is a phospholipid found in bile. It acts as an emulsifier to help break down dietary fats into smaller particles, and to help keep cholesterol in solution. Lecithin is involved in cholesterol processing in the liver, the transportation of cholesterol in the circulation and the removal of excess from the tissues. These activities depend on an enzyme called lecithin cholesterol acyltransferase (LCAT) which appears to protect against hardening and furring up of the arteries (atherosclerosis). Taking lecithin supplements has been shown to significantly improve total cholesterol levels by lowering total and 'bad' LDL-cholesterol while increasing 'good' HDL-cholesterol.

Pure cholesterol is insoluble in water, and is kept in solution within bile through interactions with bile salts, bile acids and lecithin. Lecithin supplements are therefore widely recommended to protect against cholesterol gallstones although little research has occurred in this area since the 1970s. Some early studies found that bile lecithin concentrations were lower in people with gallstones than in those without, although other studies have found no significant difference.

In one small study, eight people with gallstones took 100 mg lecithin, three times a day, for 18-24 months. All showed a significant decrease in bile cholesterol levels. One person's gallstones decreased in size and changed in shape, but no changes were seen in the stones of the other patients. This could be interpreted as a positive finding as it shows their gallstones did not increase in size or number during the study period.

Dietary lecithin is obtained from egg yolk, liver, meat, fish, wheatgerm, peanuts, Brazil nuts, beans and green leafy vegetables. The lecithin found in supplements is usually extracted from soybeans.

Dose:

A dietary intake of between 425 mg and 550 mg per day is believed to be adequate for adults.

Therapeutic doses of 2g - 4g daily are used to treat conditions such as gallstones. Higher intakes may be recommended under the supervision of a medical nutritionist.

One tablespoon of lecithin granules provides 1725 mg phosphatidylcholine and 250 mg choline – a little less than the amount present in a hen's egg. They are best taken with meals to boost absorption.

Lecithin supplements are often combined with B vitamins.

Note:
- Lecithin supplements should not be taken by those with manic depression, except under medical supervision, in case it worsens the condition.

Plant Sterols

Plant sterols (also known as phytosterols) are a group of plant hormones that include beta-sitosterol, campesterol and stigmasterol. These plant hormones so closely resemble animal cholesterol in structure that they block the intestinal receptors responsible for cholesterol absorption in the gut, although very little of the plant sterols are themselves absorbed.

A diet rich in plant sterols significantly reduces absorption of cholesterol in the small intestines, whether that cholesterol as derived from food (such as liver) or was secreted into your gut via the bile. Normally, at least 90% of bile cholesterol secreted into the intestines is reabsorbed. By consuming good amounts of plant sterols however, less of this cholesterol is reabsorbed (and recycled back to your gallbladder) as more is voided via your bowels.

Consuming 2g per day of plant sterols or stanols (similar substances derived from plant sterols) can lower blood LDL cholesterol levels by between 10% and 15% within 3 to 12 weeks - sufficient to reduce your risk of heart disease by around a quarter. Plant sterols appear to be even more effective in people with type 2 diabetes, lowering LDL-cholesterol levels by over 26% in people with type 2 diabetes, compared to a reduction of 15% in those without diabetes.

Although diet should always come first, it's difficult to obtain optimal intakes of sterols from food sources alone. The average diet provides 180 mg - 460 mg sterols per day, with vegetarians not surprisingly obtaining the highest amounts. Sterols in plant foods are naturally bound to fibre, which limits their action, however. Functional foods fortified with sterols such as spreads and yoghurts, and supplements, have therefore been developed to help boost dietary intakes.

> *Did you know?* Cholesterol-lowering statin drugs work in a different way to sterols. Statins inhibit an enzyme in the liver, so less cholesterol is made and released into your circulation. Because they work in a different way, plant sterols can be combined with statin therapy to lower cholesterol levels even further. In fact, adding sterols to statin medication is more effective than doubling the statin dose.

Increased intakes of plant sterols is one of the ways in which a vegetarian diet appears to protect against gallstones, and taking supplements might be expected to offer additional benefits to people with gallstones. Little research has been carried out in this area, however, and one widely-reported trial found unexpected, potentially negative effects with increased cholesterol saturation in those taking plant sterol supplements at a dose of 3g per day. However, what is usually not mentioned is that the fifteen patients in this trial were also taking a high dose of chenodeoxycholic acid in addition to following either a high cholesterol diet (600mg per day) or a low cholesterol diet (100mg per day). Given the small number of participants, the additional bile-modifying drug (chenodeoxycholic acid) and the dietary manipulation, it is impossible to draw any valid conclusions from this study regarding the role of plant sterols in people with gallstones.

On balance, it seems sensible to follow a plant-based diet to obtain good amounts of plant sterols from plant oils, nuts, seeds, vegetables and fruits. Good sources include olive and flaxseed oil, peanuts, soybeans and avocadoes. Sterol/stanol enriched vegetable spreads are also available as butter substitutes. If you also have a raised cholesterol level, you may consider taking plant sterol supplements to lower your risk of heart disease. There is insufficient evidence to promote their use to reduce the risk of gallstones at present.

Dose:

An intake of 1g to 3g per day is beneficial. The European Food Safety Authority (EFSA) concluded that plant sterols and stanol esters at a daily intake of 3 g (range 2.6 - 3.4 g) lower LDL-cholesterol by 11.3 % and that the minimum time required to achieve the maximum LDL-cholesterol lowering effect is two to three weeks.

Milk thistle

Milk thistle (*Silybum marianum*) has been used medicinally for over two thousand years to treat liver and gallbladder problems, including gallstones. Its seeds contain a powerful mixture of antioxidant bioflavonoids known as silymarin, of which the most active ingredient is silibinin.

Silymarin promotes liver cell function, including the secretion of bile, by maintaining levels of an important liver antioxidant called glutathione. Some studies found it boosted glutathione levels by over 33 per cent. In women, it also helps the liver metabolise oestrogen hormone more efficiently, which may also reduce gallstone formation.

By increasing the amount of bile produced, milk thistle decreases its concentration which may reduce new gallstone formation. Preliminary studies suggest it may even help to shrink cholesterol gallstones by increasing the bile acid pool, but little research has occurred in this area, and it is not possible to say how effective it is.

In the UK, milk thistle is a traditional herbal medicine licensed by the Medicines and Healthcare products Regulatory Agency (MHRA) to treat symptoms of over-indulgence, indigestion and upset stomach. Each pack therefore contains a patient information leaflet giving contraindications. It is important to read this before using milk thistle.

Dose:

Usually 100–200 mg silymarin two to three times a day (check manufacturer's instructions), preferably between meals. It is best to start with a low dose and slowly increase.

Note:
- The only reported side effect is a mild laxative one in some people, due to increased production of bile.
- Best used under the advice of a medical nutritionist if you have gallstones as increased bile flow could lead to jaundice if a stone is obstructing the bile ducts.

Globe artichoke

Globe artichoke (*Cynara scolymus*) leaves and stems contain several unique substances such as cynarin, luteolin, cynaroside, scolymoside and chlorogenic acid. These have similar liver regenerating properties to milk thistle and have been shown to increase bile secretion, improve digestion of dietary fats and reduce blood cholesterol levels.

Artichoke also contains inulin, a prebiotic fibre that stimulates growth of 'friendly' probiotic bacteria in the bowel.

A randomized, placebo-controlled trial involving 20 men with acute or chronic digestive symptoms found that taking 320 mg artichoke extracts increased bile secretion by over 127 per cent after 30 minutes, 151 per cent after 60 minutes and by 94 per cent after 90 minutes.

Artichoke has also been shown to reduce cholesterol synthesis and to lower total and 'bad' LDL-cholesterol levels while raising 'good' HDL-cholesterol. This effect is due to cynaroside and luteolin blocking the synthesis of excess cholesterol in the liver. Taking artichoke extract for 6 to 12 weeks can lower total cholesterol levels by between 4.2% and 18.5% and also reduces fatty infiltration of the liver.

Overall, its beneficial effects on digestion mean that it effectively reduces symptoms of bloating, flatulence, abdominal pain and constipation, with benefits noticed after 10 days and continuing to improve over a 6 week period.

Dose:

The usual recommended dose is 320 mg to 1,800 mg daily, with food.

Note:
- Side effects of hunger and transient increase in flatulence have been reported. Rarely, allergic reactions may occur.
- Best used under the advice of a medical nutritionist if you have gallstones as increased bile flow could lead to jaundice if a stone is obstructing the bile ducts.

Peppermint oil

Peppermint (*Menthe piperitae*) is a medicinal herb containing essential oils with both antiseptic and painkilling properties. It is used to improve digestion by increasing gastric emptying and stimulating secretion of digestive juices and bile. As a bonus, it also helps to relax excessive spasm of smooth muscle in the lining of the digestive tract – including the gallbladder and bile duct system. Some experts suggest it may help to dissolve gallstones as it has a similar profile to essential oils prescribed for this purpose (see Medical Treatments).

Although no published clinical trials have looked at the effects of taking peppermint oil alone on gallstone dissolution, private practitioners treating patients with cholesterol gallstones for six to 12 months have claimed to have seen their patients' gallstones shrink.

Peppermint oil undoubtedly reduces bowel spasm pain. A large analysis of data from 12 trials, involving almost 600 people, compared the effectiveness of peppermint oil with prescribed antispasmodics in the treatment of irritable bowel syndrome (IBS). Peppermint oil was declared the most effective medicine. On average, 75% of participants taking peppermint oil experienced a greater than 50% reduction in symptoms compared with 38%

taking inactive placebo. This suggests it's worth trying to reduce biliary colic, too.

Dose:

The usual recommended dose is 50mg to 100mg (ideally as enteric-coated capsules) three times a day, after each meal or as required.

Note:
- Treatment may produce a warm, tingling feeling in the back passage due to some of the essential oils not being absorbed. This is not harmful and will usually disappear if you cut back on the dose you are taking.
- Peppermint oil should not be taken during pregnancy.

Digestive enzymes

An enzyme is a protein that speeds up the rate at which a particular chemical reaction takes place. The 22 different human digestive enzymes you produce include:

- Proteases which break down dietary proteins.
- Amylases which digest carbohydrates.
- Lipases which break down fats.

The level of digestive enzymes you secrete depends on your genes, diet, lifestyle, gender and age.

Most people produce lower levels of intestinal enzymes and stomach hydrochloric acid as they get older, so their ability to digest and absorb key nutrients (especially B group vitamins) decreases. Lack of digestive enzymes is linked with a number of health problems including belching, bloating, wind pain, heartburn, indigestion and irritable bowel syndrome.

Many fruit and vegetables (especially pineapple, papaya, kiwi, fungi) contain enzymes with a similar action to human digestive enzymes, and can be taken in capsule form to aid digestion. Some enzyme supplements are also available from animal sources (eg pancreatic enzymes from pigs, ox bile enzyme blend that stimulates intestinal movements). Plant enzymes are usually considered superior to animal-derived enzymes as they are more stable over a wider range of acidity, and are less likely to get broken down by stomach acids.

Betaine hydrochloride may be included to promote enzyme action by boosting levels of stomach hydrochloric acid.

To improve general digestion, select a mixed digestive enzyme supplement containing lipase (digests fats), amylase (digests carbohydrates), protease (digests protein), lactase (digests milk sugar) and cellulase (digests cellulose).

Dose:

Usually, 1 to 4 capsules are taken at the beginning of a meal. Experiment to find the best dose to help your symptoms.

Check labels for 'activity units' as these show the potency of the enzymes present in a supplement. Those with the highest number of activity units are the most active.

If your symptoms do not improve within two weeks of taking digestive enzyme supplements, stop taking them and seek medical advice.

The benefits of exercise

Although not strictly speaking a nutritional approach, nutritionist usually offer advice on exercise, too. Physical activity has beneficial effects on most parts of the body, and the gallbladder is no exception.

One study looked at over eight thousand post-menopausal women and found that those taking the least physical activity were 59% more likely to develop gallstone disease than those with the highest level of activity. This was later confirmed in other studies showing that women who were most physically active were least likely to have their gallbladder removed.

For men, a study following over 45,800 male health professionals found that those engaging in an average of two to three hours of moderate running per week were between 20% and 40% less likely to develop symptomatic gallstone disease than those who did little exercise.

Although people who exercise regularly may have a healthier diet overall, there are separate reasons to explain why physical activity can protect against gallstone formation.

A higher level of sport activity appears to be associated with lower levels of bile cholesterol which would prevent cholesterol from precipitating in the bile. Research also suggests that sport activity is a more effective form of physical activity than working and leisure activities in the prevention of gallstone disease.

Overall, it appears that you need to take part in at least two hours of brisk exercise per week to significantly reduce your risk of developing gallstone symptoms that require surgery.

CHAPTER 4

Medical approaches

For asymptomatic gallstones found during routine investigation of other symptoms, the medical approach is usually one of 'watch and wait'. This is because only one in twenty-five people with 'silent' gallstones go on to develop troublesome symptoms each year.

If biliary colic develops, your doctor may treat you at home with painkillers and antispasmodic drugs if the diagnosis is certain, and symptoms not too severe. If the diagnosis is uncertain, if pain is severe, or if acute cholecystitis is suspected, admission to hospital is needed for confirmation of the diagnosis, monitoring, treatment (with intravenous fluids, antibiotics, painkillers) and assessment of suitability for surgery if indicated.

Painkillers

For uncomplicated biliary colic, the mainstay of medical treatment is painkilling drugs. An opiate analgesic called pethidine is often selected and given by injection, as it is associated with less spasm of the 'sphincter of Oddi' where the bile duct enters the duodenum. It can, however, cause nausea, vomiting, drowsiness and lower blood pressure. As a result there is a move towards using injected non-steroidal anti-inflammatory drugs (NSAIDs) such as diclofenac. Studies suggest this approach provides satisfactory pain relief for biliary colic and, due to the anti-inflammatory effect, also reduces the risk of progression to acute cholecystitis. Diclofenac also lowers pressure within the gallbladder when a stone is blocking the spiral duct (acute obstructive cholecystitis).

Antispasmodic drugs

Drugs that relax smooth muscle spasm, such as Buscopan (hyoscine butylbromide), are used less frequently now than in the past, as they appear to be less effective for pain relief than diclofenac. For example, a New Zealand study involving 72 people with acute biliary colic found that diclofenac produced complete pain relief in 92% of cases within four hours, compared with 69% with Buscopan. In addition, only 17% receiving diclofenac, which has an anti-inflammatory action, went on to develop cholecystitis compared with more than half (53%) treated with Buscopan.

Dissolving stones with medicines

The first success with dissolving gallstones medically was reported in 1972. Although dissolving your gall stones sounds like a great medical option, it is not usually that effective, and the stones often recur so you may only be postponing the need for surgery - although this isn't really a strong argument against any treatment as most people would prefer to postpone surgery whenever this is justified without increasing the risk to health.

Ursodeoxycholic acid

Ursodeoxycholic acid is a bile salt which was originally identified in polar bear bile imported from China. Its name is even derived from the Latin word for bear, which is *urso*. This bile salt was popular in Japan as a general liver tonic and soon spread worldwide when shown to dissolve gallstones.

> ***Did you know?*** *An ancient Chinese remedy for gallstones, called 'shorea' dates back to the Tang Dynasty (618 – 906 BCE). This medicine, derived from the bile of adult black bears, contained a bile acid known as chenodeoxycholic acid (CDCA). The same substance was once prescribed in western medicine to dissolve gallstones but was eventually abandoned as it raised 'bad' LDL-cholesterol and caused troublesome diarrhoea.*

Taken by mouth, ursodeoxycholic acid reduces the ratio of cholesterol to bile salts and phospholipids in bile by 40% to 60%. This allows more cholesterol to stay in solution and also dissolves some that has already precipitated out into stones.

Complete dissolution of gallstones can occur at a rate of around one millimetre (mm) decrease in diameter per month. In one study, small stones (less than 5 mm across) completely disappeared after six months treatment in around 90% of cases. The success rate with larger stones (greater than 20 mm in diameter) and multiple stones was less impressive, however, at less than 40% to 50% reduction in size after one year of treatment. This approach seems to be particularly effective for treating biliary sludge and reducing the risk of pancreatitis.

Ursodeoxycholic acid is a prescription-only treatment. Tablets, capsules and suspensions are available, but sadly, it is only suitable for treating around one in ten people with gallstones. It is licensed to dissolve small or medium-sized (less than 20 mm in diameter) cholesterol-rich (radiolucent) stones in people with otherwise normal gallbladder function. When prescribed, you will be asked to avoid consuming excessive cholesterol and calories. Your liver function will be monitored with blood tests every month for the first three months, then every three months. Tests to check the progress of gallstone dissolution are also needed every six to ten months.

Unfortunately, gallstones usually recur (because of the genetic and dietary factors that caused them in the first place) in one in four patients within one year of stopping treatment. Other studies have reported recurrence rates of 30% to 50% within five years, and up to 70% within 12 years of initially successful treatment. That does, however, mean that at least 30% of those suitable for treatment remained gallstone free after 12 years without needing to undergo gallbladder surgery.

Contraindications

Ursodeoxycholic acid cannot be used if you have calcified (radio-opaque) stones, a non-functioning gall bladder, acute inflammation of the gall bladder (cholecystitis) or biliary tract, frequent episodes of biliary colic, or if you have inflammatory diseases or other conditions affecting the liver, small or large intestines. It should not be used in pregnancy, breastfeeding, or if you may become pregnant.

Side-effects

Common adverse effects include mild diarrhoea and 'pasty' stools; very rarely abdominal pain, gallstone calcification, nausea, vomiting, itching and allergic reactions have been reported.

Dose:

Usual dose is 6 to12 mg/kg body weight per day, either as a single dose at bedtime or in two divided doses. Typically, 450mg to 600mg is prescribed. This may be increased to 15mg/kg daily if needed. Treatment is continued for up to two years, depending on the size of the stones, and for 3 to 4 months after the stones have dissolved.

Terpene essential oils

A mixture of terpene essential oils (borneol, camphene, cineole, menthol, menthone, pinene in olive oil) is available on prescription (as Rowachol) to raise bile cholesterol solubility and help dissolve gallstones. It also relaxes the bile ducts and may help to reduce painful spasm of bile ducts and the expulsion of gallstones. However, its use is in decline and the British National Formulary states that it is 'not considered to be a useful adjunct.'

Interestingly, peppermint oil contains a similar level of menthol and menthone as Rowachol.

Rowachol is licensed for the management and dissolution of cholesterol (radiolucent) gallstones in people with a functioning gall bladder. There are no known contraindications, but it is not normally used during pregnancy or breastfeeding.

This mixture of essential oils stimulates bile production in the liver as well as reducing the formation of cholesterol crystals in bile. It has also been used to enhance the effectiveness of bile salt treatments such as ursodeoxycholic acid. Clinical trials suggest treatment can completely dissolve gallstones in 29% of cases at six months, 37% at twelve months and 50% after two years.

Some doctors may consider using Rowachol to dissolve cholesterol stones in the common bile duct where surgery is not feasible. However, in one series of patients, more than 25% of those treated still developed biliary colic, obstructive jaundice, pancreatitis or cholangitis (inflammation of the bile duct).

Dose:

Usual dose is 1 to 2 capsules, three times a day before meals.

Statins

Statin drugs (eg atorvastatin, fluvastatin, lovastatin, pravastatin, rosuvastatin and simvastatin) are widely prescribed to lower cholesterol levels. They work by blocking an enzyme (HMG-CoA reductase) which is involved in the synthesis of cholesterol.

Taking statins for at least five years reduces the risk of coronary heart disease (CHD) and stroke by around one third. Initially, they were only prescribed for people at high risk of coronary heart disease or stroke because of a raised cholesterol level. Then, in 2002, the Heart Protection Study which involved over 20,000 people, showed that statins appeared to reduce the risk of these events in everyone, even those with an ideal total cholesterol level of <5.0 mmol/l. There did not seem to be a lower cut-off for cholesterol levels beneath which the benefits ended.

The decision to prescribe a statin is therefore no longer based on your cholesterol level alone. Statins are recommended for anyone whose likelihood of developing CHD over the next 10 years is 20% or greater. This risk is calculated from charts, based on your gender, age, smoking status, blood pressure, cholesterol levels and whether or not you have diabetes. The general aim of treatment is to lower your LDL cholesterol to <3.0 mmol/l and your total cholesterol to <5.0 mmol/l, or by 30%, whichever is greater, but the decision to prescribe a statin is no longer based on your cholesterol level alone.

Recently it was recognised that statins also have potential as a treatment for cholesterol gallstones. Statin treatment has been found to reduce bile cholesterol levels and, in some cases, to dissolve cholesterol gallstones

A US study involving around 121,700 female nurses found that statin use reduced the risk of needing a gallbladder removal by around 12% compared with non-users. Interestingly, statin users had more risk factors for gallstones than non-users (eg diabetes, being overweight, exercising less, smoking more) which might suggest the protection level is even higher.

Did you know? *Statins also block synthesis of an important cell nutrient called co-enzyme Q10.*

If you are prescribed a statin drug to lower your cholesterol or reduce your risk of heart disease, it is important to know that statins also switch off production of co-enzyme Q10. This may be one of the underlying causes of the muscle aches and pains experience by a significant number of people taking statin medication. In fact, a patent filed for the first statin drug suggested that it should be given together with CoQ10 supplements to prevent these muscle side effects, although this was not acted upon.

Co-enzyme Q10 is needed for energy production and is especially important in muscle cells, including those in the heart. When CoQ10 levels are low, cells cannot produce adequate energy, function less well and are more likely to become diseased. Biopsies from people with various forms of heart disease have shown, for example, that between half and three-quarters are deficient in CoQ10.

While statins can reduce cholesterol levels by 40% to 50%, they also reduce CoQ10 by the same amount – and often more quickly. In fact, taking a statin can halve your circulating blood levels of CoQ10 within just 2 weeks. Although lowering CoQ10 levels may not cause problems for healthy volunteers, it can worsen heart problems in some people.

Did you know? Statins sold in some countries, such as Canada, carry a warning that they may seriously deplete CoQ10 levels in *the body, which can lead to impaired cardiac functioning in people with congestive heart failure.*

Importantly, taking co-enzyme Q10 supplements maintains blood levels of CoQ10 without affecting the cholesterol-lowering action of the statin drug. A recent study showed that combining simvastatin with 60mg CoQ10 produced improved heart health benefits compared with taking simvastatin alone.

Doses:

The dose of statin drugs differ across the range, and depending on response, from 5mg to 80mg daily.

Co-enzyme Q10 in the ubiquinone form is typically taken in a dose of 200mg for those on statin drugs; Co-enzyme Q10 in the ubiquinol form (more readily absorbed and used in the body) –is typical taken at a dose of 100mg.

CHAPTER 5

Surgical Approaches

The surgical approaches used to treat gallstones include shattering with shock waves, and gallbladder removal (cholecystectomy) which can be carried out via laparoscopy (keyhole surgery) or via a larger abdominal incision.

Lithotripsy to shatter gallstones

In 1985, extracorporeal shockwave lithotripsy (ESWL) was first used in Germany to shatter bile duct stones that could not be extracted using an endoscope. This technique uses focused shock waves (produced using electromagnetic or ultrasound sources) to fragment gallstones and is sometimes used in combination with oral medical treatments such as ursodeoxycholic acid to dissolve the fragments produced.

The main disadvantages of lithotripsy are the need to instil a cholesterol solvent into the gallbladder or bile duct to dissolve the fragments (otherwise they would trigger pain while being passed) and the high recurrence rate of up to 26% within two years. It is not therefore not widely available or used except in elderly patients who are not fit or well enough to undergo open surgery.

Gallbladder removal

Cholecystectomy – the medical term for removal of the gallbladder – was first carried out in 1882 and is now one of the most common abdominal operations. Traditionally, it involved a large up-and-down laparotomy incision, which was later refined to a smaller cut beneath the ribs on the upper right-hand side of the abdomen. These open operations were considered major procedures and carried significant risks.

Then, almost a hundred years later, everything changed in 1987 when the first laparoscopic (keyhole) cholecystectomy was performed in France. This minimally invasive technique has transformed the safety of gallbladder surgery and remains the first-choice for surgical treatment of gallstones. However, according to the National Institutes of Health in the US, it is important that its availability does not expand the indications for gallbladder removal. Gallstones that are not causing symptoms do not usually warrant gallbladder removal as the risk of gallstone-related complications is rare without having at least one episode of biliary pain beforehand. The wait-and-see approach is still recommended.

At one time, surgery was postponed if cholecystitis was present to give your gallbladder time to recover. However, this can lead to adhesions (scar tissue) forming internally that makes removal more difficult. Research now shows that removing the gallbladder early during an episode of acute cholecystitis leads to quicker recovery and a better outcome than the traditional approach of waiting for six weeks until the inflammation settled down.

What happens during gallbladder surgery?

Your surgeon will explain the planned procedure with you, and discuss the possible complications as well as the benefits. Write down the things you want to know before the consultation so you remember to ask. Once you decide you are happy to proceed with surgery, you will sign a consent form to show you understand the risks involved.

Your surgeon or anaesthetist should ask about any medicines, over-the-counter remedies or supplements you are taking, as some may affect blood clotting, or interfere with anaesthetic drugs. If you are not asked, volunteer the information, as you may need to stop taking them for a week or more before surgery.

Sometimes surgery is scheduled quickly, but it is common to wait a few weeks or even months. Use this time to ensure you are as fit as possible before surgery.

Any excess weight you can lose will help the surgeon and reduce your risks of complications. If you smoke, it is vital to stop. Smoking cigarettes increases the risk of abnormal blood clots, impairs healing and lowers your immunity so you are more likely to experience an infection.

Before the operation

For a general anaesthetic, you will usually be nil-by-mouth for at least six hours (or overnight) beforehand. One to two hours before surgery you will receive medication known as the 'pre-med'. This usually includes a drug to reduce anxiety and help you relax (important to stop your blood pressure going too high), an antacid plus drugs to reduce salivary secretion and nausea. You may also be asked to wear graduated compression stockings to reduce the risk of blood clots developing in the deep veins or arteries of the legs.

Laparoscopic cholecystectomy

A laparoscopic cholecystectomy typically takes between 45 minutes and one hour. Once the general anaesthetic kicks in, you are moved onto a special radiolucent operating table (through which X-rays can pass) so that imaging studies (cholangiography) can be performed.

A nasogastric tube is then passed down through your nose to empty any stomach juices present. This ensures no stomach acids are pushed up into your throat when air is pumped into your abdominal cavity, and a catheter inserted to empty your bladder.

Step 1: The surgeon makes an incision in your umbilicus (belly-button) and inserts a tube to pump air into your abdominal cavity. This pushes your intestines out of the way and lifts your abdominal wall to give the surgeon a better view.

Step 2: A laparoscope (camera) is then inserted through this initial incision and the surgeon checks all your abdominal and pelvic organs to rule out any unforeseen problems such as adhesions.

> *Adhesions are fibrous strands of scar tissue that form within the abdominal cavity as a result of previous inflammation or surgery. They may form thin strands or a dense web over the surface of internal organs so that, for example, the gallbladder becomes matted to the liver. The risk of developing adhesions increases with age, episodes of cholecystitis, and with the number of previous abdominal operations you've had. Adhesions increase the total time of an abdominal operation, as they obscure the normal anatomy so the surgeon needs to carefully cut them away.*

Step 3: The operating table is tilted slightly head up and sideways towards the left. This lets your intestines fall away from the liver so the surgeon can get a clearer view of your gallbladder. This is essential to ensure it is safe to proceed.

Step 4: Typically, the surgeon makes three further small incisions in your abdominal wall. One incision is usually at the top of your abdomen just below the ribs, and close to the gallbladder. The position of the remaining two incisions in the lower abdomen vary. Some surgeons make two incisions in the lower right abdomen, while others make one on the right and one on the left.

> *Did you know?* A new technique that uses only one incision in the umbilicus (single-port cholecystectomy) was developed in 2008 and is becoming more popular. A special device containing three separate access points is inserted into this single incision through which all the necessary surgical instruments are inserted and manipulated. Ask your surgeon which technique and incisions he favours.

Step 5: Forceps are passed through one hole (or the single port) to grasp the top of your gallbladder, another set of forceps are passed through a second hole (or port) to grasp the neck of your gallbladder, and the surgical cutting instruments are passed through the third hole (or port). If you have a 'floppy' liver lobe which obscures the surgeon's view, another incision may be needed to insert a retractor which holds the liver back.

Step 6: The surgeon grasps the main pouch of your gallbladder with blunt forceps and pushes it up over the front of the liver, towards your diaphragm, as far as it will go. If the pouch is very distended with trapped bile, sludge or stones, it is drained with a needle and syringe and the contents sent to the laboratory to look for any infection that needs antibiotic treatment. If your gallbladder has previously been inflamed (cholecystitis) the surgeon may need to separate strands of scar tissue (adhesions) to separate the gallbladder from your liver using a hot probe (diathermy).

Step 7: The surgeon now grasps the neck of your gallbladder with another set of forceps and looks for an important anatomical landmark between your liver, the cystic duct (leading from the gallbladder) and your common hepatic duct. Known as Calot's triangle, this area contains your cystic artery which supplies blood to your gallbladder. If this area is difficult to identify, either because of fatty tissue, scar tissue or unusual anatomy, the surgeon will abandon the laparoscopy and proceed to an open operation for your own safety.

Step 8: The surgeon carefully teases out your cystic artery and cystic duct and seals them using titanium clips, absorbable clips, or loops of suture, depending on the surgeon's preference. Around this time, the surgeon will usually perform an intra-operative cholangiogram.

Intraoperative cholangiography

The link between your cystic duct and gallbladder is first sealed off with two clips (insurance in case one slips off). An opening is then made in front of the clips and the tip of a catheter inserted into the cystic duct and held in place. A 'dye' is injected through the catheter to outline your biliary duct system. Originally, the dye was designed to show up on X-rays but it is now more likely to be analysed using real-time fluoroscopic imagery, which provides immediate images without the delay needed to develop X-ray films.

Intraoperative cholangiography shows the surgeon your exact biliary anatomy (some patients have unusual accessory ducts or even two gallbladders) and whether or not you have a gallstone lodged in your biliary duct. As many as one in ten patients with no symptoms of a common bile duct stone do actually have one and, if identified now, this can be dealt with during the operation rather than causing problems afterwards. Cholangiography performed during surgery only adds an extra five minutes to surgery time and is becoming routine. Studies show that patients who've a cholangiogram during surgery are less likely to have their bile ducts injured during surgery as any unusual anatomy is known before the surgeon starts cutting into the area.

Step 9: Your gallbladder is now carefully trimmed away from your liver using scissors or a hot knife. The surgeon will check to see if you have an additional small bile duct leading from the liver into the gallbladder (bile duct of Luschka) in which case this is sealed and clipped, too.

Step 10: When your gallbladder is fully separated from your liver, it is held to one side with forceps and the underlying liver bed is washed with saline. This will reveal any bleeding points that need to sealing, either with heat (diathermy) or stitches.

Step 11: Now comes the clever part. The surgeon inserts a moistened retrieval bag through one of the abdomen incisions (or an umbilical port) and holds it next to the detached gallbladder. The forceps holding the gallbladder and its contents is now manipulated to tuck the removed organ inside. The retrieval bag is then sealed, so no bile, gallstones or sludge can leak out, and removed through one of the incisions. If a gallstone is too large to pull out, it is simply crushed within the retrieval bag to avoid having to enlarge the incision.

Step 12: After retrieval of the bag, the surgeon has a final look round to double-check for bleeding or bile leaks. You may have a long-acting local anaesthetic injected into the sides of the wounds to reduce post-operative discomfort. Your abdomen is then emptied of as much air as possible to reduce post-operative discomfort, and the incisions are closed with sutures, tape or staples. Some patients may have a drain left in place overnight to check there is no bile leakage, but this is not routinely needed.

Your gallbladder will be sent to the pathology lab where it is examined under a microscope to exclude any unexpected abnormalities such as a gallbladder cancer. If you would like to keep your gallstones as a memento, let your surgeon know. Where possible he will wash and retain them in a specimen pot for you to take home.

If your recovery is routine, you can usually go home on the day after surgery providing there are no complications.

Open cholecystectomy

Sometimes an open cholecystectomy is planned from the start (for example if you have cirrhosis of the liver, are pregnant, or if there is a suspected cancer). Usually, however, a surgeon will first attempt a laparoscopic cholecystectomy and only convert to an open operation if difficulties arise. There is a low threshold for conversion as this is not seen as a failure of surgical technique, but simply as safe practice. Reasons why a surgeon may decide to switch to an open operation include:

- Poor view - especially in people who are very overweight.
- Unclear or difficult anatomy - it's estimated that only one in four people have what is classed as 'normal' anatomy of the gallbladder and bile ducts. One in 4500 people have two gallbladders!
- The presence of internal bands of scar tissue (adhesions) from episodes of cholecystitis or previous abdominal surgery.
- Bleeding that is difficult to stop.
- Anything that causes the surgeon to feel it's unsafe to continue with a planned laparoscopic cholecystectomy.

Conversion to an open operation occurs in between one in ten and one in a hundred procedures. It is least likely when uncomplicated gallstones are present, and most likely if you have acute cholecystitis when the chance rises to one in five. Surveys show that patients most likely to proceed to an open cholecystectomy have one or more of the following factors:

- Age 60 or more.
- Male.
- Weigh more than 65 kg.
- Have acute cholecystitis.

- Have had previous upper abdominal surgery.
- Have diabetes, especially if it is not well controlled.

What happens during an open cholecystectomy?

An open cholecystectomy often only requires a short incision (5cm long) in what is called a mini-laparotomy. Sometimes, however, a longer incision of 15cm is needed to gain access, especially in larger patients.

Step 1: The surgeon cuts through your skin and the subcutaneous fat and muscle layers beneath. Small bleeding points are sealed with heat (diathermy) with the surgeon taking care not to burn your skin. If a larger blood vessel is cut, it is closed with a fine absorbable suture.

Step 2: The sides of the incision are held back with expandable retractors. The surgeon carefully picks up a fold of the peritoneal membrane which lines your abdominal cavity, using toothed forceps. After ensuring it is not stuck down to adhesions, bowel or an inflamed gallbladder, the membrane is cut to expose your abdominal cavity.

Step 3: Any adhesions are carefully lifted with tissue-holding forceps and cut. This requires patience, as the surgeon must always clearly identify what he is cutting before using a scalpel, scissors, or hot blade (diathermy) to avoid damaging any underlying structures. The operating table is tilted slightly head up and sideways towards the left, so your intestines fall away from the gallbladder under the influence of gravity. This gives the surgeon the best view of the operative field.

Step 4: The surgeon carefully examines your abdominal organs by feel and, where possible, by sight, to exclude any unforeseen diseases or other problems. This examination is carried out in a methodical order using the same sequence each time, so nothing is missed. Moist packs are inserted to protect your liver and intestines and push them out of the way.

Step 5: The surgeon now takes time to identify Calot's triangle - an important anatomical landmark between your liver, cystic duct and common hepatic duct. Difficulty identifying this anatomical triangle is a common reason for having converted from a laparoscopic to an open cholecystectomy. Calot's triangle contains the cystic artery which supplies blood to your gallbladder.

Step 6: The surgeon cuts and seals both the cystic artery and cystic duct, then performs an intraoperative cholangiogram to visualise the anatomy of your biliary ducts, and to check whether or not there is a 'silent' gallstone in your common bile duct.

Step 7: The gallbladder is cut away and removed. The underlying liver bed is washed with saline and any bleeding points sealed with heat (diathermy) or stitches.

Step 8: Once all bleeding has stopped, the surgeon may rinse your abdominal cavity with warm saline. If bleeding or bile leakage has occurred, or is suspected, a drain is inserted which will be removed after 24 hours if it remains clear. The incision is then closed using the surgeon's preferred method – some like to stich each layer separately, while others prefer one simple closure of all except the skin which is stapled or sewn separately, and the wound is dressed.

An open cholecystectomy may take from one and a half to three hours. You will usually need to stay in hospital for four to five days afterwards.

Avoiding future adhesions

It was recently realised that the starch powder used to coat latex surgical gloves so they are easier to put on may trigger adhesion formation. Thoroughly washing the gloves for 10 minutes, after putting them on, may reduce adhesion formation. Another option is for a surgeon to use powder-free gloves. Rinsing the abdominal cavity with a solution known as Ringer's lactate at the end of surgery appears to inhibit adhesion development. As sewing the peritoneum can also trigger adhesions, many surgeons now avoid this, too. Some use adhesion-prevention barriers made from cellulose or Gore-Tex to line surfaces where adhesions commonly form.

So that's it, really. I have included in this guide all the useful information I could find to help you overcome your gallstones, whether you prefer a nutritional approach, need to take medicines, or are contemplating surgery. I hope you have find it helpful. If so, please consider providing a review on Amazon.

Best wishes for your future good health, Dr Sarah Brewer.

Bibliography

Some of the sources used while researching this Help Yourself Guide include:

www.ncbi.nlm.nih.gov/pubmed A comprehensive searchable list of medical research papers.

Acalovschi M. Cholesterol gallstones: from epidemiology to prevention. Postgrad Med J 2001;77:221-229

Atamanalp SS et al. The effects of serum cholesterol, LDL, and HDL levels on gallstone cholesterol concentration. Pak J Med Sci 2013;29(1):187-190.

Behar J et al. Functional gallbladder and sphincter of Oddi disorders. Gastroenterol 2006; 130:1498-1509

Gaby AR. Nutritional approaches to prevention and treatment of gallstones. Altern Med Rev 2009; 14(3):258-267

Guarino MPL et al. Ursodeoxycholic acid therapy in gallbladder disease, a story not yet completed. World J Gastroenterol 2013; 19(31): 5029-5034

Reshetnyak VI. Concept of the pathogenesis and treatment of cholelithiasis. World J Hepatol 2012; 4(2):18-34

Tsai CJ et al. Statin use and the risk of cholecystectomy in women. Gastroenterology 2009; 136(5):1593-1600

Walcher T et al. Vitamin C supplement use may protect against gallstones: an observational study on a randomly selected population. BMC Gastroenterology 20099; 9:74

Dr Sarah Brewer's previous books include:

Nutrition: A Beginner's Guide, OneWorld, 2013

Eat Well, Stay Well, Connections, 2013

Live Longer, Look Younger, Connections, 2012

Death: A survival Guide , Quercus, 2011

Cut Your Stress, Quercus, 2010

Essential Guide to Vitamins, Minerals and Herbal Supplements, Right Way, 2010

Cut Your Cholesterol, Quercus, 2009

Natural Health Guru: Overcoming Arthritis, Duncan Baird, 2009

Natural Health Guru: Overcoming Asthma, Duncan Baird, 2009

Natural Health Guru: Overcoming High BP, Duncan Baird, 2008

Natural Health Guru: Overcoming Diabetes, Duncan Baird, 2008

Diabetes Cookbook for Dummies, Wiley, 2007

Menopause for Dummies, Wiley, 2007

Thyroid for Dummies, Wiley, 2006

Arthritis for Dummies, Wiley, 2006

Natural Approaches to Diabetes, Piatkus, 2005

Intimate Relations; Living and Loving in Later Life, Age Concern, 2004

The IBS Diet, Thorsons, 2004

Daily Telegraph Complete Guide to Menopause, Robinson, 2003

Eat to Beat High Blood Pressure   Thorsons   2003

Live Better: Relaxation, Duncan Baird, 2003

Encyclopaedia of Vitamins, Minerals & Herbal Supplements, Robinson, 2002

1001 Facts about the Human Body, Dorling Kindersley, 2002

Energy Boosters Handbook, Dorling Kindersley, 2002

Eat to Beat IBS, Thorsons, 2002

A Child's World (Channel 4 series), Headline, 2001

The Total Detox Plan, Carlton, 2000

Simply Relax, Duncan Baird, 2000

Saw Palmetto – Natural Prostate Relief, Thorsons , 2000

Pregnancy – The Natural Way, Souvenir, 1999

Increase Your Sex Drive, Thorsons, 1999

I Want To Have A Baby?, KyleCathie, 1999

The Ultimate Stress Buster, Vermilion, 1998, 2003

Super Baby, Thorsons, 1998

The Osteoporosis Prevention Guide Souvenir, 1998

Man Alive: Eating Fit, Marshall Ed, 1997

Man Alive: Better Sex, Marshall Ed, 1997

Menopause, Thorsons, 1997,

Candida, Thorsons, 1997,

Irritable Bowel Syndrome, Thorsons, 1997

High Blood Pressure, Thorsons, 1997

Body Facts Pocket Guide, Dorling Kindersley, 1996

Endometriosis and Fibroids, Vermilion, 1995, 1998

Beating Heart Disease the Natural Way, Galen, 1995

Factopedia: chapter on Human Body , Dorling Kindersley, 1995

The Complete Book of Men's Health, Thorsons, 1995, 1999

Planning a Baby? , Vermilion, 1995, 2004

The Hypochondriacs' Dictionary of Ill Health, Headline, 1994

The Body Awareness Programme, Bantam, 1994

What Worries Women Most, Piccadilly Press, 1993

The Bluffers' Guide to Sex, Ravette, 1987-2014

CPSIA information can be obtained at www.ICGtesting.com
Printed in the USA
LVOW04s1511030415

433204LV00014B/300/P

9 781500 806767